MAKE. A. PLAN.

THE REAL-WORLD GUIDE
TO KICKING ASS
AFTER WEIGHT LOSS SURGERY

BY

CHRISTY BAILEY

CONTENTS

FOREWORD

As I sit down to write this little gem, we are in the midst of the whole COVID-19 disaster. Like so many others in the country, I find myself with free time that I had to fill with something. See, I tried filling it with food, but when my pants got tight, I thought, *put down the cookie and do something productive with your quarantine, woman.* I give myself pep talks all the time. You should try it.

Really, though, I saw myself picking up some old habits with my eating when the boredom, stress, and fatigue set in. I had gastric sleeve surgery a couple of years ago and a few pounds have crept back. Everybody on Facebook is talking about eating to cope, and baking, and complaining about getting fat during quarantine, and it made me feel okay about eating junk. Everybody else is doing it, right? Then I put on my shorts from last year and was like, nope. Party's over. It's time to make a plan.

I am a 43-year-old wife and mom, travel agent, writer, and fitness junkie, and I love the control I have finally gained with my surgery. I like meal prepping and cooking healthily for my family, and I also love making cakes for them and enjoying ice cream from my favorite snow cone stand. I love the balance of life. I'm the "in the middle" gal. Queen of moderation. I tried all that when I was 240 pounds. It didn't work then. Now it does. Hallelujah! I love to research and organize and plan things, and I have helped friends figure out macros to fit their goals and helped them with workout plans to fit their life, so I thought, why not put it into a book?

I know there is a growing number of us that have had weight loss surgery, and my heart breaks for those who aren't having the long-term success they want. Maybe by helping them, I will also help myself to avoid those same pitfalls.

This book will be intentionally concise and short. If a self-help, diet, or strategy book is too long, I tend to not finish it, and I'm that person who loves to read and plan. So no, it will not be long, but it *will* be jam-packed with info to get you on your way. It will have forms to help you plan and track your progress.

You've been warned. I am not a doctor. I am you. I've been in the trenches and I've fought the fight. I live in the real world. I'm not going to tell you to eat a can of tuna with fat-free mayonnaise and be happy. Hell, no. I'm going to show you how to eat smart and still enjoy life. I'm gonna teach you how to work out without becoming a gym rat (unless you want to become a gym rat, because I am totally a gym rat). And I'm going to teach you how to harness the power of the pouch. All of these will be baby steps in a six-week program to get you back on track.

CHAPTER 1

HERE'S WHAT IT'S ALL ABOUT

So Here You Are

For years you were overweight. You struggled for so many years of your life to manage it and be healthy. You fought it. You gave up. You started again on Monday. You succeeded a lot, but you failed more. Sound familiar? Low-fat, Jenny Craig, Weight Watchers, Atkins, macro-counting, keto. You went into each diet so sure that this was it. This diet would finally fix you. You joined a gym, yoga, lifted weights, walked for miles, CrossFit ... Some things stuck; some things didn't even last a week. Then one day, you hit this wall. You hit it hard and just collapsed and said, "I give up." Then something shifted and instead of giving up, you just shifted your thinking. You changed courses. You made an appointment, and you started the process to have WEIGHT LOSS SURGERY, right? The light at the end of the tunnel. Months pass and then years, and then you come out the other side. You heal, you eat less, you shed the pounds, and you're now magically cured. Problems over. The end ... right? WRONG.

Whether you have had a gastric bypass, gastric sleeve, gastric band surgery, or any other type of surgery to help you lose weight, the other side is relatively similar for all of us. Success and failure vary from one person to the next, and there's still work to be done for most of us. (By the way ... I'm a sleeve gal!)

Most post-weight loss surgery patients fall into one of two categories:

UNICORNS: These are the people who even years after surgery are still at an ideal weight. They don't even have to count calories, they're not particularly concerned with exercising, and the portion control the surgery brings is enough to keep them perfectly on course. This is the outcome most patients expect to have, but honestly, it's rare.

WORKER BEES: This more common category is where a lot of us fall. We lost the weight as predicted and thought we had this thing licked! Then, as the years pass, we realize that maybe we aren't living a fairy tale after all. Some of us are able to recognize this early and do enough to manage things. Maybe our weight fluctuates from five to eight pounds depending on the time of the year. Not too shabby. We spend a certain amount of time counting calories, jogging, following the rules, but with this new "tool" we've been given, we can finally make things work for a change.

Another group of us maybe saw those pounds coming back but weren't able to get a handle on it. The five pounds became ten pounds became twenty pounds. Every Monday we vow to start again, and suddenly we feel plunged right back into the person we were before surgery. But there's hope. They don't call us Worker Bees for nothing.

Whether we find ourselves two pounds higher than we want to be or sixty pounds higher than we want to be, we can climb our way back. We have this new practical tool in our bodies (aka a teeny tiny pouch instead of a stretchy balloon of a stomach) that we just have to learn to manage—or relearn to manage in some cases. You just have to take the first step, adopting one simple change and making it a new habit and then tackling another one. Again and again. Nothing drastic and nothing crazy. Just commitment to small change. Harnessing the power of the pouch.

Yes, I had the gastric sleeve years ago, and yes, I'm in the WORKER BEE category. I am having success for the time being, and here's why: I had some good habits going into the surgery. I am sure you're wondering why someone with good habits needed surgery to lose weight. Believe me, I've analysed it again and again, and that is ANOTHER book entirely, so let's just stay on topic, people.

#

What Got Us Here

I am going to be straight with you. I am a 43-year-old woman who has evolved and changed and tried very hard to learn and be better over the years. The years have brought with them a major pet peeve, and it revolves around complacency. More specifically, complaint paired with complacency. To be blunt, I take issue with people who bitch and complain about something, but literally do nothing—NOTHING—to change it. I know change is hard. I get it. I don't doubt it for a second. I know most of us, including me, can't or won't just flip a switch and change everything, but we CAN change small things.

Here's the deal. If you are truly not happy with something—your weight, your relationship, your financial situation, your mental health, your career, your loneliness, your child's behavior, your gray hair (geez, I could go on and on)—if there is something in your life you are not happy with, for God's sake, make a plan to change it. Break it down into baby steps and start the journey. Your happiness and well-being are completely in your own hands. That's it. Whatever happened in your past, whatever is holding you back, is now your responsibility. Make a plan, ask for help, take some action. Don't wallow in it. Do. Something. Stop blaming the world and other people and do something. Make. A. Plan.

Some people might say, "That's big talk from someone who gave up and had surgery to lose weight." First of all, sit down. Second of all, I did not give up. I moved on to plan B because plan A wasn't working. I quit beating my head against a wall and feeling sorry for myself and took action. I do that in all areas of my life. I don't ever give up, but I may find a new way to get there. That's what successful people do.

If I just bummed you out, I'm sorry. The fact is, when presented with a problem, my mind goes straight into problem-solving mode. I don't know why. And I often don't understand why others don't think the same way. It's my strength, but it is also my flaw.

On a positive note, reading this book—or any book that will help you, for that matter—is the start of change! So maybe you didn't need that lecture. I'm preaching to the choir, as they say. Bravo to you for taking that first step. You're already leaps and bounds ahead of lots of other people. You see a problem. You are doing something about it. Here we go.

Let's just go ahead and list some of the reasons we MAY be gaining weight after surgery:

You stretched out your pouch. It can happen. That cute little pouch can apparently stretch a bit, but in my personal experience and from what I learned during my research and by talking to other weight loss patients, I don't feel that this is the main problem. For sure, people who continuously overeat to the point of painful fullness, again and again, are bound to stretch their stomachs, but even those who can consume more than the ideal amount still cannot consume large enough amounts to derail their weight loss. You still can't eat as much as you did before surgery. Also, according to my doctor, the portion of the stomach left behind after surgery is the thicker, less flexible part of the stomach that would be very difficult to stretch out without chronic, persistent overeating. So, there's that …

You are not getting enough exercise. Most people don't exercise enough, and I mean MOST PEOPLE, not just the curvy people in the world. I absolutely feel that exercise is one of the keys to weight management, but it does not take the top spot. From my own experience, before and after surgery, exercise, though important, is not the answer. It's just part of the answer.

You are eating too many calories. Ding, ding, ding. We have a winner. It's not really a shocker, is it? Even a tiny pouch can hold a lot of calories. You know what can fill a pouch from top to bottom comfortably? Ice cream, chocolate, movie popcorn with extra butter, mashed potatoes. These are just four of the endless calorie-dense items that melt down and conform perfectly to a tiny area. The drastic weight loss in the beginning lulls us into this confident state that tells us to enjoy ourselves because we're part of the thin crowd now. We fall back and embrace what is familiar.

It's so simple, but it's so complicated. Are these the only reasons? No. It is more than likely a combination of these reasons. Do we have to factor in other reasons that aren't even listed above? Yes, we do. These are just the broad categories that give us a guideline and a map to figure out a path forward. They help us Make. A. Plan.

Here's the thing: knowing the problem is one thing, fixing it is another, but all things are possible. One thing that won't fix the problem is sitting around, being sad, and complaining. No, we were not born the lucky ones with super high metabolisms. Yes, we do have to work harder than most. Everybody has problems and obstacles they have to work through in life. Many people out there have far greater problems to struggle through than carrying extra weight. This is our burden, and we can face it and start taking small steps toward success, or we can just accept our fate. The choice is entirely ours.

DISCLAIMER: So, you've gained some weight. I bet you are still beautiful and/or handsome. I bet you are still smart and talented and loving. If you are happy with yourself and want to embrace your curves and not be bound by societal norms, by all means just live your life and be happy. I am dead serious. Curves are sexy, and everyone, male or female, deserves to live in whatever body they want.

If this does not pertain to you and you find your weight limiting you from what you love doing, then proceed. I love to hike and bike with my family and I don't want to be slowed down. I also don't want to slow them down. I love to jog and want to do it without blowing out my knees. I want to know I can fit in any roller coaster because I *love* roller coasters. I don't want my sleep apnea to return because someday soon I want to climb Machu Picchu. I want to camp in a tent without worrying about a CPAP machine. If you are like me and you want to do better (and I am assuming you do because you bought the book), then do the next right thing to move toward something better. Don't. Be. Complacent. Make. A. Plan.

#

Warning Signs (let's get this out of the way)

Before we proceed, let's discuss some true warning signs that reveal bigger problems, problems that this book can't truly help with. Gaining some weight is one thing. This is common and just means it's time to get smart and be cautious but not be overly worried. It's not easy, but you can fix it with a little guidance and some determination and hard work. But we need to talk about the other situations some of us find ourselves in post–weight loss surgery. These incidents occur when people were maybe not emotionally ready for this huge life change called weight loss surgery but had it anyway. These are the people whom doctors attempt, or at least should attempt, to weed out, or at the very least offer further guidance and education before performing the procedure. They attempt to do this by sending us to nutritionists and therapists beforehand. It is why having a good doctor is so important; you should not be able to decide to have this major surgery and then have it a month later. This lack of forethought and planning is one of the reasons we got into these overweight bodies to begin with. Let's take a hard look at some warning signs. If you identify with any of these situations, you probably have an issue that needs more help than my little book can offer.

Stomach pain after eating. Guys, if you're eating so much that your stomach is hurting after meals, you have a problem. I'm not talking one meal now and again, because we all get too full occasionally. I'm talking to those of you having significant pain after many meals. You're overeating to the point of major discomfort. You're eating too fast, and your brain can't catch up until it's too late. You're putting too much food on your plate to begin with and then lingering over it after you're full ... nibbling. These are signs of addictive behavior, and you truly need someone to help you one-on-one. A therapist may need to give you the special attention you need, the tools to take care of yourself. It would take fifteen minutes to go online and find one to text with, so quit being a scaredy-cat and face your demons. YOU are DEFINITELY worth the work and DEFINITELY worth the money.

Vomiting. If you are pushing so far past the point of fullness that you're barfing, we have a major issue. If it happened once and you learned your lesson, that's one thing. If you're doing it every weekend, it's bad, my friend. You have developed an eating disorder. You know it's bad, and I know it's bad. If seeing it written down and reading it helps to get your brain to now register the seriousness of this, then good. Go find some help. If you are this obsessed with food, you need personal guidance. Bite the bullet and find a therapist. There are better ways to live your life than letting food control you.

Laxative abuser. You know that this is just another form of an eating disorder. Sure, we all use a little help now and again when things aren't working right and the system comes to a halt. A little MiraLAX, some fiber, sometimes the occasional laxative, but not on the regular. If you're using it to "detox" or to "cleanse" after a binge, you know it's a seductive habit. You probably also know that it doesn't really do any good or help with long-term weight loss. Throw them into the trash, drink some water, eat some veggies. That's how you cleanse. If you are buying and using laxatives more than once a month, stop and get some help. If you're doing this, I can bet you're having some of the other issues we already discussed, like overeating and possibly vomiting. It's time for therapy.

Drinking too much. Most of us like to have a little drinky drink on the weekends. You may even have an occasional girls' night where you get wasted. Hey, I'm not advising it, just saying it happens (in my case, about every three months or so). But if you're drinking daily (more than a glass of wine with dinner) or you're getting wasted every weekend, you're getting into dangerous territory. Addictive behavior is a common trait among overweight individuals. Doctors are seeing a rise in post-weight loss surgery patients becoming addicted to things other than food. Suddenly there's this hole in your life where food used to be, and some people need to fill it. Some people use alcohol, some use sex, and some use drugs. I wish I could just say stop and tell you how to replace drinking with exercise or knitting. If only it were that easy. If you feel yourself becoming more reliant on alcohol to fill the empty void in your life, you are not alone. You also need major help, but you have to recognize and ask for it. Don't waste your new life being wasted.

Drugs. I don't care if you have a prescription or buy it from some guy down the block. If you are abusing any type of drug to cope with life, you need help. Look, I'm not talking about anti-depressants here. I'm not even talking about Xanax or Klonopin if you're using it appropriately. But if you are taking a prescription drug like Xanax, Klonopin, pain pills, etc. and you feel like it has more power over you than you have over it, you definitely need some help. And if you're using anything illegal, then it goes without saying. Run, don't walk. You've come this far. Are you going to let this ruin your life? Because it's only a matter of time if you don't do something about it. Get help!

I hope most of you skimmed over this section because it did not apply to you at all. Sadly, I have personally seen these issues plague people after their surgery. When you can no longer cope by using food, you turn to other things. If any of these things are going on in your life, don't hesitate to ask for help. Moving on ...

CHAPTER 2

MENTAL GAME

What Motivates YOU?

When each of us made the decision to undergo major surgery, we had a list of reasons in our head, or maybe even on paper, as to why we were taking this major step. Some would even consider it a drastic step. Do you remember what yours were?

I resisted surgery for quite a while, and I actually quietly judged others who went that route. I thought they had given up and/or not tried hard enough. I was wrong, of course. I suppose some people didn't try hard enough, but it still wasn't my place to judge. What actually planted the first seed in my mind to consider weight loss surgery as an option was a meal with my best friends. We were sitting around a dinner table and discussing this person or that person who had undergone weight loss surgery. I should interject here so you don't get the wrong idea. We were discussing a certain individual who we knew for a fact had had gastric bypass surgery. This person also kept this information on the down low. No problem. Your business ... except that we often heard him telling people things like "When are people going to learn it's all about a lifestyle change?" or making people believe that his weight loss was nothing beyond exercise and a good meal plan. It was deceptive and cruel to say something like that to a group of women (I witnessed it) that he was training—women who were working hard to be healthy with normal gastrointestinal systems. He could have just as easily motivated them by saying, "Yeah, I had the surgery, but I still work hard to stay this way and stay healthy" or something along those lines. We were in a gym when I heard his comments and I almost fell off the weight bench. Be upfront or don't say anything. I would never want someone out there working hard to lose the weight thinking "The CrossFit is finally paying off for Christy. If only I would get off my ass, I could finally lose the weight too." It's not always that simple, and I would never want to mislead anyone or have them think less of themselves.

So, back to the dinner with friends. Keep in mind that none of these friends sitting at that table with me had ever dealt with any serious weight problems, at least not on the same level as me. One of them asked me, "Christy, you would never consider surgery?" I wasn't insulted, because at 240 pounds it was a valid question. My answer was something like, "I couldn't exercise like I do now eating so few calories." You have to understand that I was doing CrossFit, and I felt strong and I loved it so much. The basic response from my friends was "Just know that we would never judge you if you did. We've watched you work harder than the rest of us for years and we want to see you succeed." They probably have no idea how floored I was. Not offended or hurt at all, just floored that I hadn't considered it sooner. I realized that the only reason I hadn't was because I didn't want to be the pitiful person who had to have surgery. I didn't want to be "fake" like the person we had been gossiping about. The seed was planted, though, and for the first time I considered that I could have the surgery and still be genuine and real with people.

The seed grew over the next year. I realized also that I had rejected the idea of surgery because I didn't want to lose weight just for vanity's sake. Meaning, I didn't want to have it just to look a different way. If I was living the life I wanted, physically and mentally, I couldn't see a valid reason to have major surgery. I was teaching my daughters to accept their bodies, be healthy, and not let other people tell you how you should look, so I wanted to be the best example I could be for them. How could I tell them to be comfortable in their own bodies and not try to be like what they see on television when I was willing to have surgery to look a different way? That was how I saw things. I didn't want to be a hypocrite.

Then I took a hard look at my life. I was starting to have knee problems. I couldn't hike as fast as my family could or enjoy it as much as them. I had developed sleep apnea that was almost certainly caused by my weight. Was my quality of life as good as I claimed? My husband and I really do want to travel and hike up mountains with llamas and sleep in tents next to Sherpas. Between bad knees and a CPAP machine, that wasn't really a possibility. It was time to face the facts. My body was holding me back from more than I realized.

So, my motivation to stay light, agile, and healthy is so I can be active with my family and husband. I love to travel, and I plan to travel much more as our children leave the house. I don't ever want to hold my husband back or limit my own life. Plus, I love to exercise (I know, I'm a weirdo). I love seeing the new things my body can do now that it is lighter.

Now it's your turn. Why did you have the surgery? Maybe your reasons were similar to mine. Maybe you were more interested in wearing cuter clothes or wanting to feel more confident in a bathing suit. Look, I didn't have the surgery for that specific reason, but I get it. I love not going into the plus-sized section anymore. I love sharing some clothes with my daughters. So if you had it for "vanity" reasons, you won't get any judgment from me. You do you!

It is time to revisit your original reasons for major weight loss and maybe add some new ones to keep the weight off. Take a minute to think back and write down the reasons.

WRITE AT LEAST 3 REASONS YOU HAD SURGERY. Be as specific as possible.

1._____

2. _____

3._____

4._____

5._____

Here's my list.

1. To be able to hike up a mountain and camp out without dying or blowing out my knees.
2. To be able to continue to work out hard without damaging my body in the process.
3. To kick sleep apnea's ass and throw my CPAP in the garbage (I did, by the way).
4. To finally end the cycle and struggle of weight loss once and for all.
5. To not let my weight ever hold me back from any adventure I decide to pursue.

Don't cheat and steal mine ... I'm joking; you can steal one if it works for you. Sometimes putting pen to paper and writing it down really solidifies something inside of us. We need to remind ourselves of the reasons we took this huge step, because they are the exact same reasons that we want to keep that weight off. They're the same reasons we need to lose weight again. Stop wasting time and take this small second step. The first step was buying a book, so congratulations, but I'll wait here while you go grab a pen from the junk drawer. Don't convince yourself you'll keep reading and come back to fill in the blanks. You won't. Go get a pencil from your kid's backpack. Use a lipliner. Don't make excuses. I'll wait ...

Are you back? You have a writing instrument? Bravo, my friend! Bravo! Think and write. Think deep thoughts and write them down.

#

Mental Strategies

As we continue down the mental path, let's discuss your options for support and strength to get you through the challenges. You may have noticed we are not going to talk about fitness first, and we aren't going to talk about food yet. That is because we are getting in your head first. That should tell you how important this step is. Let's talk strategy.

Mental Strategy #1: Find a teammate who wants to be healthier.

Significant other. Your boo is the best place to start, especially if you live together or are married. You guys need to be on the same page, at least as far as food goes, because if not, somebody is gonna be pissy. Either you, as you watch them eat thick crust pizza without any regard for your goals or happiness, or they may get a little petty if they're not mentally prepared for grilled asparagus, ground turkey, spaghetti squash, and organic sugar-free pasta sauce. You get the idea. They can be your best ally or your worst enemy. Get 'em on board.

Your best friend. Maybe they need to shed a few pounds too, or at least adopt a healthier lifestyle. Let's face it. Most people want to lose a few pounds or at least get healthier.

Your mom or dad. Parents are always there to support us, no matter how old we are. Or that's how it should be. They can be your afternoon walk partner, Sunday dinner planner, or they could be someone to text when you're having a bad day. Moms and dads tend to be either positive or matter-of-fact, and either one is handy in this situation.

A co-worker. If you work, then there's a good chance you've bonded with someone at the office. You can plan meals together, remind each other to get that water in before lunch, and they can go for a walk with you while you drink meal replacement smoothies together.

Your child. You would be surprised how excited some kids get about being healthy, especially if they know that they're helping you. Whether they are nine years old or nineteen years old, they could all do with some healthier habits. They typically have tons of energy, which is great motivation. They will also bug the ever-loving crap out of you until you go jump on the trampoline like you promised.

Mental Strategy #2: Join a group.

Facebook group. This does not have to be a group dealing only with gastric surgery lifestyle. This could be any healthy eating, positive thinking exercise group that feels right to you. These could be people in your community or people across the country. If you can't find one that suits you, start one yourself. Invite people that you know want to be healthy and you guys can support each other from afar. You can share motivational posts, sweaty workout pics, workout suggestions, or recipes.

Group chat. This is more personal. This is a group of like-minded friends all texting within the same conversation. There are four of us in my group chat, and these are my besties. They all like to exercise, even if it's just a little. We all like to motivate each other, and our husbands all get along. We get together as often as possible, but we literally text the group on and off all day, always post pics of our daily workouts, and often send pics of our food logs at the end of the day when we were all working hard. It is a mental game changer! We also talk crap about people who annoy us. We vent about our husbands' back hair and how loudly they chew. We talk about how cute/annoying our kids are. This group chat is crucial to my life. Period. Get one started.

Support group. There are some of you who are not interested in Facebook or texting and are much more comfortable with face-to-face situations. So be it. I suggest asking around or possibly talking to the doctor's office that performed your surgery and asking if they are aware of any support groups in your area. Another version of a support group is **Weight Watchers, or WW** as they're referring to themselves now. I liked the weekly Weight Watchers meetings I used to attend back in the day, even if I did nothing else but weigh and leave. Even if you're at your ideal weight, you can join for the purpose of maintenance. Check online and see if there's one in your area. They even probably have a number to call if that's more your speed. I just spent five seconds on my phone and found the number: 1-800-651-6000, so no excuses.

Mental Strategy #3: Get professional help.

Find a real-life therapist. This is not an easy task for some people. Personally, I worried about finding the RIGHT therapist for ME. We always worry about being judged. Luckily, I did meet a helpful one, which my surgeon set up for me because it was required by my insurance. He was kind and knowledgeable and I haven't felt the need to revisit him, but it is nice to know I have the option. To meet regularly with a professional who can give you advice and insight into your issues would be invaluable to someone struggling.

Find an online therapist. Okay, so this concept is sorta new, but it interests me. I am a bit of a homebody, and introverted, so texting back and forth with someone feels like a more realistic option for someone like me. If this interests you, a good option seems to be betterhelp.com, which provides individual, couple, or teen counseling. They offer video, phone, live chat, and messaging. There is also talkspace.com, which offers all the same communication options. These are just two of many choices out there, so if your time is limited or if you're like me and feel that starting the therapy process online is less intimidating, you should do some research and give them a try. All help is welcome when you're trying to reach goals.

Mental Strategy #4: Keep reading and keep learning. Reread and relearn.

This book. You're reading this handy little guidebook, so ... yay, you! Take notes, use the worksheets, make a plan. Strategize. What has worked before? What didn't? A year from now, after the holidays, or after some backsliding, pull it off the bookshelf and read it again; remind yourself why getting back on track and staying focused is important to you.

Do more research. Whether it's a TED Talk on YouTube where someone is discussing the finer points of reaching goals or a Netflix documentary about organic farming, learn what makes people healthy. Browse Pinterest or Amazon and find other books that deal with the same issues. The therapist I visited before my surgery recommended a book called *The Beck Diet Solution*. It is a six-week strategy to train your brain to think differently about food and your body and how to create better habits. It is practical and slow paced, and it was one of the many steps of learning that helped me gain success.

Noom. I'm not sure what category this should fall under, but I feel like, even though it is a weight loss app, it should be mentioned under the MENTAL heading because it uses psychology along with a meal plan to help you reach goals. Much like *The Beck Diet Solution* book I mentioned, it deals with how to make small changes in habit and thinking to shift you to better decisions and success. If you already know what to eat and how to exercise and are still struggling, this may be an app to consider. It has a two-week free trial before you commit, then it costs $59 a month unless you sign up for an annual membership, which is $199. Try it for two weeks and see if it works for you. If so, then the fee is worth it if it gets you heading back down the right path. Am I right?

Podcasts and blogs. I am a podcast nerd. I would rather listen to a book or a podcast than listen to music. It drives my family crazy. If you haven't gotten on the podcast train, let me indoctrinate you. There are podcasts about EVERYTHING. Literally. So, you guessed it, there are even podcasts for people who have had weight loss surgery. Podcasts often bleed over into blogs, which bleed over into Instagram accounts, which overlap into Facebook accounts. Just search "weight loss surgery podcasts" and see what happens. Again, you don't have to limit yourself to things that fall under the "weight loss surgery" banner. Any weight loss system or advice can be beneficial.

CHAPTER 3

FITNESS

Exercise ... Sorta the Answer to EVERYTHING

Here's the deal: I worked out consistently and I worked out hard for six years before I had my gastric sleeve surgery, and I definitely lost weight here or there, but it is NOT the magic key to weight loss. Is it important? Absolutely, but do you have to become a gym rat or join CrossFit or start running 5Ks to get the benefits? No. Is it fun to do all those amazing things? Yes ... for some people.

Consistent exercise has many benefits, and we all know this. It has been proven to help prevent many things, from heart disease to cancer to diabetes to mental illness; it also prevents bone loss and muscle loss as we age. So many benefits. These few factors I listed are a good enough reason for you or any other person to make an effort to be a bit more active in your daily life.

When my husband turned forty and I turned thirty-six, we woke up one morning and my husband said, "Damn I'm old," as he slowly got out of bed. He rubbed his shoulder and rubbed his back because they bothered him all the time. I looked at his belly and I looked down at my own and said, "We're not old. We're just fat and out of shape, babe." I had pretty much had enough, so, like many wives do, I took charge and decided we were going to join an Anytime Fitness that had just opened in our town, and we even hired a trainer. Best. Decision. Ever.

We both agreed (he came around) that the least we could do for our bodies was to exercise. Even if we still ate fried chicken and drank Cokes (or sodas or pop for you northerners) every day, we would at least get our workouts in. The money for the memberships and the trainer was money well spent. It truly started us on the path to taking care of ourselves. It also grounded our relationship because of this shared commitment and new shared hobby. Our lives were forever changed. It was actually that trainer (thank you, Rhonda Bradley) who told me that if I wanted to stick to an exercise habit, it had to be a commitment to health and not just weight loss, because everybody jumps off the diet wagon eventually. It's human nature. Exercise needed to be the constant. She told me then that weight loss was 20 percent exercise and 80 percent diet. I had no idea.

When exercise becomes a habit, do or die, you won't just get those amazing health benefits; it is also a reminder to do better. When you jog, or pick up a dumbbell, or do yoga, you're reminding yourself that your body is special and important, and those thoughts carry over into the rest of your day. Because you did that mile walk or maybe because you did those fifty push-ups on your lunch break, you will make more and more healthier decisions like eating the grilled chicken instead of the fried, or eating that orange at three o'clock instead of the honeybun. People who work out consistently make healthier decisions in all other aspects of their life.

So, to recap, exercise is not the answer, but it is part of the solution.

#

Choosing What Works for You ...

But I don't know how to work out. I don't know what to do. Elliptical or treadmill? Dumbbells or machines? Zumba or yoga? What is the best?

The best thing is whatever you are willing to do ... for at least twenty minutes three to five days a week. PERIODT. (My daughter taught me that. Look it up.) You should start with whatever gets you excited ... or whatever makes you cringe the least. You do not have to become an athlete overnight. As a matter of fact, you do not have to become one at all. You just have to move in whatever way appeals to you on a regular basis. Just move with some purpose. Let me get you started.

WALKING. Walking, people. It is literally the easiest option. It requires no training, no experience, no warmup, no cool down. Everybody can find thirty minutes in their schedule three to five days a week. You don't have to join a gym or plan a workout to get started. You don't have to walk five miles, or jog, or even walk fast. Just set aside thirty minutes, put on some comfy shoes, and put one foot in front of the other. You can take the dog, you can take your kid, you can push a stroller, you can take your neighbor. You can walk in the mall, you can walk outside and look at the trees, and you can even walk in the rain, which I actually love to do sometimes. You are getting health benefits, and you're getting that all-important reminder that your body is valuable and you should take care of it.

STRENGTH TRAINING or CARDIO TRAINING. These are just broad terms that cover many areas of fitness, but basically strength training is a focus on muscle toning and muscle building versus cardio training, which focuses more on building your endurance and lung strength. Many people do a little of both on any given day. Some people alternate strength training days with cardio training days. Some people do weeks or months of mostly strength training and then spend the next few weeks doing mostly cardio. Some people do workouts (CrossFit, for example) that do both at the same time, which is super effective but also really overwhelming for some. Imagine your lungs burning and your biceps burning at the same time.

Which one is best for weight loss? There are many schools of thought and many different opinions, but truly the answer is whichever one you enjoy or are willing to do on any given day. There is no right answer and there is no wrong answer. They both burn calories, they can both raise your metabolism, and they both benefit your health. Periodt. (Did you look it up yet?)

Cardio training is less intimidating to most people and is the best place to start. Get on a treadmill. Get on an elliptical. Get on a bike. Go for a walk. Go for a jog. Row. Whether you're in a gym or outside, these are easy options that don't require much more than just getting going.

Strength training can require a little more planning and has more of a learning curve, but it is also not that complicated. Whether you're using machines at the gym or dumbbells at home, a plan to follow is just a click away. You can buy a book with diagrams and pictures. Pinterest has tons of workouts to get you started. YouTube has a billion videos with people like me demonstrating proper bicep curls, how to get a rounder butt, and how to tone your back. If you're willing to look, there is tons of information out there for you, most of it free.

HIRE A TRAINER. If you've never met a trainer, you're probably imagining some muscled-up person in a tank top who likes to torture people. That may be the case sometimes, but mostly they're just regular people who like working out and like getting paid to help people. They rock. If you can afford it, do it! You'll learn you're probably gonna show up because you've paid for it, and you will probably make a lifelong friend. And if they turn out to be a muscled-up person in a tank top who is mean to you, you can just break up with them and go for a walk instead.

A FUN FITNESS CHALLENGE. This is just a variation on the standard workout you may find online, and the simplicity of a **thirty-day challenge** is appealing to a lot of people. If you don't know what it is, just type "fitness challenge" into a search bar and you'll see endless options. I'll say it again … Pinterest. Seriously, though, if you're not on Pinterest on the regular, you're missing out big time. These challenges usually last for thirty days, and the movements are often simple, like push-ups, sit-ups, lunges, planks. One may be walking a certain number of miles in a month. Most of these challenges will be short, simple, and sweet and require little time out of your day, but the benefits will add up. It's a no-brainer! Someone has already done the work, typed it up, and it's there for anyone to use. You can share it on Facebook or Instagram and drag a few of your friends or co-workers on board. Keep this in mind, though: these challenges should be a launchpad into something long-term. Remember to have a plan in place as to what is next for you before those thirty days are up. If you're not sure or the challenge is over and you haven't made a decision, it's no big deal. Just go back to filling your time with walking until you find another challenge that seems fun.

VIRTUAL RACES. I have recently learned about virtual races, and it's my new favorite thing. If you go online and look, you will see so many options, and many of them raise money for charity. You basically sign up and pay, committing to a 5K, a 10K, a marathon, or my husband and I actually opted for a longer race lasting forty miles. They're based on the honor system, obviously, because no one would be the wiser if you actually ran a 5K or not. When you're done, you get your medal and/or T-shirt in the mail. Ours is a Yes.Fit **(yes.fit.com)** race, and we chose the Yeti one, which is the same distance as a hike through Nepal. It will take us a month or so to get all the miles in to complete it, but it gives us a new, fun motivation to get that extra mile in. Each time you add your workout, it shows you pictures of where you would be on the actual hike, and since we love to travel, we just eat it up. You have to keep things fun.

GOOGLE IT. Literally, people. There are a million and one ready-made workouts just sitting there ready to be printed out. Hello! Pinterest! If you haven't already learned the usefulness of Pinterest in your life, you will when I'm done with you. Just type "quick workouts for beginners" into the search bar, close your eyes, and choose one. You can't go wrong. You could also be one of those people who makes a post on Facebook that says, "I need an easy workout, guys ... And go!" and make other people do the work for you, but I really don't like those people. Hello! Pinterest! Weight-lifting workouts, couch to 5K workouts, living room workouts ... so many options.

Remember to keep moving! Remember you're not only burning calories; you're reminding yourself that your body is important and you have to take care of it.

#

Tips and Tricks: Fitness

So, along the way I have picked up a few things, as well as seeing what is working well for other people.

If you look good, you feel good. This goes for girls and guys. Some cute workout clothes go a long way to keeping you motivated, whether it's how you feel when you put them on or the significance of laying them out in the mornings and seeing a visual reminder of what you expect from yourself. Having said that, if your workouts are small and concise and happen in your bedroom ten minutes before you hop into the shower and you'd rather do them in your jammies, I get it. But if cute clothes help keep you motivated, then go with it. You have my permission, and I talked to your parents/husband/wife/accountant and they said it's okay. Buy the cute leggings.

Suggestions

Old Navy (oldnavy.com). I wear workout clothes pretty much every day because I work out in the mornings and I work from home, so I'm too lazy to change. Old Navy supplies most of my gear. They're affordable, you can shop online, they have plus sizes, they have tall, they have petite, and they look freakin' awesome. Trust me, if my booty can look good in them, anybody's can.

Lululemon (lululemon.com). Some people swear by Lulu and refuse to wear anything else. I get it. They're cute. They make your body look good. They are high quality. They are a little pricey for me, but I don't judge. If it gets you moving, then go get you some.

Find a partner. This is sometimes hard because the majority of people out there are not consistent when it comes to exercise, and they will most likely be harder to lure off their couches as the weeks pass, but just keep trying and eventually you will find a teammate. This could be your teenage daughter, your hubby, your wifey, or even your lesbian neighbor who already has a Bowflex. It could even be your office mate who is willing to walk with you to Subway and back for a tuna sandwich. It will probably be your dog after a few weeks, but that is totally fine. Maybe you like to work out alone. If so, you still need someone who is willing to work out often so you guys can brag to each other and motivate each other. You can keep each other accountable by sending each other red-faced sweaty pictures after workouts or pics of your Apple watch proving you burned calories.

Suggestions: Find any freakin' body who is consistent and who will keep you excited about getting that exercise in. If all else fails, adopt a dog that loves to walk.

The worst thing you can do is overdo it. Yeah, you heard that right. Pace yourself. I would rather see you adopt a workout plan in the beginning that is ten minutes a day five days a week than see you join a gym and workout for two hours every day. The first one is doable and sustainable, and the latter one is likely to either burn you out or give you an injury. If you go from watching Graham Norton clips on YouTube every afternoon to running a mile in a week, you are gonna get plantar fasciitis, a swollen knee, or both. I know because I am guilty of that. Slow and steady wins the race. Baby steps. Consistency is key. After thirty days of doing ten-minute workouts, your attitude will be "No big deal, I can do another month of this." After only seven days of crazy two-hour sessions, you will say, "F&6k this. I'm tired and I hate my life."

Suggestions: Start small and be consistent.

Get good shoes. This applies to you guys who plan on doing a lot of walking or high-impact stuff. Suck it up and get a great pair of shoes that are right for your feet. Just spend the money. If you walk a lot, be prepared to replace them regularly. Getting a foot injury like plantar fasciitis is terrible, so try to avoid it. It can be hard to get rid of and can seriously slow down or stop you in your tracks. Your feet deserve nice shoes. The right shoe will depend on how high or low your arch is. It may also depend on whether your feet roll inward, outward, or not at all. A specialized shoe store usually has employees that can assess the right type of shoe for you. If there isn't one in your area, you may have to do your own research.

Suggestions: Fleet feet (fleetfeet.com) is an athletic shoe chain and the one in my area was able to help me find a good running shoe. My favorite brand is (saucony.com), and they have an online questionnaire to help you find the shoe for you (www.saucony .com/en/content?caid=shoe-advisor). My daughter's favorite is **Brooks** (brooksrunning.com), and they also have an online questionnaire to help you find the right shoe for you (www.brooks running.com/en_us/ShoeFinder).

Make. The. Time. You don't have time to work out ... Umm, sorry, but I don't believe you. If you have time to scroll on Facebook or you have time to walk through Bath and Body Works and lift the lid of every one of those candles and sniff them, then you have twenty minutes to spare on your body. If you work eighty hours a week at a desk with no breaks, then get a standing desk, do some squats in between emails, and do standing push-ups off the copier while it makes your copies. It's all possible. But seriously, it may mean getting up earlier than usual, which sucks, so lay out those gym clothes the night before. They'll be staring at you when you open your eyes in the morning. You can do it. It may mean heading to the gym after work, which also sucks, so pack those cool workout clothes into a fancy new gym bag the night before. Go put it in your car before you go to bed. Put it in the front seat, so you don't forget. It may mean doing your thirty-day fitness challenge in your cubicle in your work clothes because you know you're gonna crash as soon as you get home. You've got this!

Suggestions: This is where the worksheets I provide will come in handy, because planning is a must. I can't solve this one for you; you have to find that time somewhere. Plan your life, or your life will plan you. Plan your day, or your day will plan you. Replace a timewaster (I do have a Pinterest problem at times) with something more useful. Make it happen.

Anything can be modified. You can't do a push-up? No big deal. Do them on your knees. Still too hard? Do ballerina push-ups, where your pelvis stays on the floor (google it). Do you have bad knees? Bad back? Google "workouts for people with bum knees" and you'll learn plenty. If you do have some limitations, don't let it stop you. Talk to your doctor and work on a remedy. Another great way around this is hiring a trainer. They are going to be able to work around those problems. It's their job. There are legit 85-year-old people still working out, so you can too!

Suggestions: It comes down to excuses at this point. Worst-case scenario, you have a big enough health limitation or injury preventing you from exercising that requires you to talk to your doctor. Okay. Go talk to your doctor. Together you can make a plan that's safe. Any workout can be modified for any age or capability if you're willing to put in the work.

#

For Example, ...

So, you want me to hold your hand? Fine ... this can get you started.

Workout 1: Set a timer for 10, 15, or 20 minutes and repeat the following cycle as many times as possible until the timer goes off.

- 5 air squats

- 5 push-ups

- 5 sit-ups or crunches

- 5 jumping jacks

- You don't have to rush; just nice slow, steady movement.

- Do it Monday, Wednesday, and Friday and try to get better every time.

- After a couple of weeks, try doing 10 of each movement, etc.

Workout 2: Tuesday, Thursday, and Saturday go for a 30-minute walk.

Workout 3: Go outside and set the timer on your phone for 20 minutes.

- Walk around for a bit and then stop and do some lunges.

- Walk around some more and then stop and do some burpees.

- Walk around some more and then stop and do some squats.

– Walk around some more and then stop and do some push-ups off a tree.

– Continue until timer goes off.

Are you getting the idea? You can literally start anywhere! Don't make it complicated unless you're ready to make it complicated. Will this get boring after a while? Probably. I suggest you find something that makes you happy. Zumba classes are fun. Maybe a hip-hop step aerobics routine works for you. Maybe you still cling to the Cindy Crawford workout that you did twenty-five years ago (my mother does), which is totally great. As long as you're doing stuff, you're good.

CHAPTER 4

FOOD

FOOD ... Now We're Getting to the Heart of the Matter

We've all had our stomachs shrunk, or had our insides rerouted, or had a section pinched off, so food isn't an issue anymore, right? Not so fast. Most of us find out after a certain period of time that we now have a helping hand, but we don't have the magic bullet to long-lasting weight loss. The fact is, many of us found ourselves overweight and needing weight loss surgery because we more than likely had an unhealthy relationship with food beforehand. It's sad, but it's true. Many of us, at the minimum, had some bad habits that we may not have corrected before going under the knife. The good news is, if you're struggling with weight gain post-surgery, you stand a much better chance of managing it now than you did before the surgery. You now have a great tool to help you get a handle on things, but you have to do your part and you have to learn, plan, and put in the work.

First of all, we need to realize that what works for one person doesn't work for everybody. Some people, including doctors, think they have everything figured out.

"If you just ate fresh food ... preservatives are killing us."

"It's calories in, calories out ..."

"Carbs are the enemy ... Sugar is the devil."

"Not all carbs, just complex carbs are bad ... Eat all the veggies!"

"If you just eat six small meals, you will raise your metabolism ..."

"If you just fast for certain periods, you will raise your metabolism ..."

"High fiber ..."

"High protein ..."

We have heard all these things. Especially, you hear it from the person this one plan has worked for and this person swears it's the answer for you too. They'll swear they've cracked the system! But no, the fact is, there are many routes to get to the same place, and it isn't a one-size-fits-all situation. Sometimes it doesn't work for one person for psychological reasons, meaning it's just not a good fit for their likes, dislikes, or lifestyle. Sometimes it really is a chemical thing, meaning that for whatever reason, what causes one human to lose weight just doesn't work for another human. For example, I've done the low-carb thing and for sure I lost weight, but it only took me so far. Eventually, I had to also cut calories and/or fat too, or I wouldn't lose any more. I would just plateau. My husband, on the other hand, would shrink down to gristle if he could just avoid carbs. Also, and I'm about to be very blunt here, unlike many others on a low-carb diet, it gave me terrible diarrhea. The forums online all said it was temporary and that it would get better. No, it wasn't, and no, it didn't. It was terrible. And psychologically, low-carb is difficult for the long-term. It's kind of an all-or-nothing situation, and who wants to avoid cake at a birthday party FOREVER or chocolate FOREVER? Okay, maybe not forever, but even most of the time without those things sucks big time. And don't tell me sugar-free is good too. No, it isn't. And sugar-free stuff can also give you ... diarrhea.

The fact is, different plans work for different people. Some need structure, or it will never work for them. Some people need flexibility, or it will never work for them. The trick is finding the one that works for you.

#

Portions

Let's take a moment to discuss portion size. If you are at least a year out from surgery, you should be thoroughly healed and ready for the long haul. Your portions at this point are going to vary depending on what you're eating. For example, I can eat about a cup of something soft like cottage cheese, yogurt, ice cream, or chocolate. But if I eat something denser like chicken, a protein bar, or steak, I find that I can't quite get the same amount in. You can see why our food choices still greatly affect our weight loss and maintenance.

Most people, believe it or not, are not gaining back their weight because they have stretched their stomachs back out. The bigger problem is often WHAT they are eating and HOW OFTEN they are eating. Having said that, if you feel that your portions have grown larger than you would like, then let's stop to think about what small changes need to be made to correct it.

Slow the hell down. Quit eating so fast! Slow down and thoroughly chew your food. Imagine you're trying to get it to the consistency of applesauce before swallowing. Talk to your family in between bites. They're not home? Talk to your cat in between bites. Put your fork down while you're chewing. Savor the food. You might as well, because our meals are tiny these days. You should truly be mentally present and fully appreciate your small portion. Plus, when you're out with friends and finish eating way before everybody else, it's kinda awkward. This step is key, because if you eat quickly, you're more than likely going to get too full, and you're going to get there before you even realize it. You're going to consume fewer calories if you give your body time to tell you you're full. Slow the hell down.

Quit drinking with your meal. This is standard advice we are given post-surgery. I assumed originally that this was because we would fill up with liquid and not be able to get enough food in to be healthy. I later learned that it's the opposite. Drinking can sometimes flush the food through faster; therefore, you may eat more at that meal, or you get hungry soon after eating. In my experience, it does not affect my portion size at all when I drink with a meal, but perhaps it's because I only take a few sips. I also don't feel that I get hungry sooner, but EVERYBODY IS DIFFERENT. For the sake of learning, commit to no liquids with your meal and see what happens.

Choose protein first. This is a no-brainer that we know we should do but don't always follow through with. Your plate has two ounces of grilled chicken and a quarter cup of broccoli and rice casserole (your momma's recipe made with butter). Which one do you eat first? I should say, which one SHOULD you eat first? You should eat the damn chicken first with just a tad bit of casserole mixed in. Don't opt for only the casserole, because (a) it's calorie dense, and (b) it's weak on protein. So, you've eaten lots of calories and you'll be hungry in a hot minute. That's no good. Be smart. Eat mostly chicken with a little bit of casserole.

Any of these three options—eating slower, no drinking with a meal, and choosing protein first—are great goals on their own. If you're not ready to adopt a new diet and don't want to exercise at all, then that is okay. When we get to the plan, you'll see that this is our only goal in the beginning. We're going to pick one of these simple changes and commit to it for a week. We're gonna use your tool the doctor gave you (I'm talking about your tiny pouch). The next week, we'll make a new goal. Add another small change. These are basic, bare-bones, no-excuse ways to get back on track. These small changes could make a huge difference. If you did one or all for only one week and lost one pound, that's a great payoff for very little effort and definitely worth a try!

No one is suggesting you completely overhaul your life if you're not ready. JUST PICK A SMALL GOAL AND DO IT!

#

Pouch Reset

Some people feel that this should be step one if you've gained a decent amount of weight after weight loss surgery. They feel that a pouch reset is necessary because their pouches have just stretched too much over time. No offense, but chances are, they're wrong. My surgeon told me that the part of the stomach left after surgery is thick and tough and not prone to stretching. Stretching only happens for some people if they are overeating meal after meal, day after day. If this is you, I think you need more learning and structure than a five-day pouch reset can offer. Even so, if a short pouch reset seems like something that will get you back on track, then follow your gut. It feels a bit like a crash diet, which we all know is bad news, but if it helps reset YOUR BRAIN, then go ahead and push the reset button.

The basics. If you do a little googling you will find some simple five-day or ten-day pouch reset diets. Basically, you go back to liquids for day one, then soft foods for day two, then progress to more regular food, similar to post-surgery. If you're trying to "detox" a little to get off caffeine, sugar, or gluten, then maybe this will help. You do you.

Be careful. Don't set yourself up for failure. This will take some planning. A stocked fridge is necessary, and be prepared to take food everywhere you go—broth, Jell-O, protein shakes. If you last two days and then binge on pizza, did you do yourself any favors?

If things don't go as planned. If you find yourself too weak to function properly, if you find yourself angry at people around you for mocking you with their chewing while you slurp broth, if your angry little pouch growls so loudly that you can't hear the television, then geez ... regroup and reset. Eat some chicken. It's okay. A liquid diet was tough when my stomach physically rejected anything else. Doing it with a perfectly functioning tummy, even a smaller one, is kinda like torture. There are so many options that can get you back on course without suffering. Don't go overboard. Don't beat yourself up. None of us is perfect. When we fail at one thing, we don't give up. We move on and ask ourselves, "What's next? That didn't work, so what else can I do?" You keep looking for the path. You don't give up.

#

To Track or Not to Track

So, what am I talking about? I'm talking about tracking your food. You know, that tedious thing where you write down everything that goes into your mouth on a given day. It can be aggravating, it can be time-consuming, and it can also be necessary ... at least for a little while. It is the only way you're really going to know where things are going wrong. A bite here and a bite there add up. A handful of M&Ms that you ate out of your kid's bag when they weren't looking, or that sweet tea you drank ... those things that you think don't matter really *do* matter.

It's time for a reality check. You do not have to commit to tracking food 100 percent of the time. I don't. You go back to tracking when you need to, and you wing it when things are going well. If you're reading this book, then things are not going as planned. Honey, it's time to track. I'm not even saying you should change your eating yet. Eat like you normally do and keep a journal. You might be surprised. Don't think ignoring it will help. Just suck it up and face the music.

Here are some ways to track:

Pen and paper. Literally just grab a notebook and something to write with. If you bite it, you write it. You may want to buy a nice notebook to remotivate yourself. Maybe something leather, maybe something with sparkles, or whatever floats your boat. A little splurge that reminds you that you're committing, or recommitting, yourself to eating healthily. A fancy pen, perhaps ...

My Fitness Pal app. This is my go-to. It's free, it's easy, and you know you have your phone with you at all times anyway. The database is huge, so if you type in, for example, Wendy's chicken nuggets or homemade apple pie, there will be options. You even have the ability to scan the barcodes of items or put in your own recipes.

Weight Watchers app or WW. This one costs money, but if you're willing to join, I think it's a great option. I would still suggest you give the My Fitness Pal app a try before committing to WW, though.

After a few days, look for a pattern. You can look back over a few days of tracking and the problem should be clear. You're probably going to see that your calorie intake is way higher than you realized. Or if you're a low-carb person, you're going to see that your carb intake crept up higher than it should be. If you look back and don't see a problem, then maybe you adjusted your usual eating because you knew you had to write it down. Cool. Give yourself a pat on the back and keep tracking. That's kinda the whole point.

#

Pick a Plan, Any Plan

If you haven't figured it out yet, I'm not that person who is going to tell you which plan is best. Sorry. The fact is, I don't know which plan is best for you. I'm afraid you are going to have to figure that out, but I'm going to help you out. Here are some of the basic plans that are out there right now, and they are all plans I have personal experience with. And I'll also explain why each tends to work for us (us being people who now have tiny little pouches).

LOW-CARB

Why this works for us: The fact is, when our portions shrink after weight loss surgery, we have to be careful to take in enough protein. Why is protein important? If fills us up and keeps us full for longer than carbs. It also helps to maintain and build muscle, which is important for our health and metabolism. A low-carbohydrate diet naturally leans toward protein sources, which is a good practice for people after weight loss surgery. You get your protein, you stay full, problem solved. Yes ... and no. If it works for you, then yay! Tracking food becomes much easier and maybe unnecessary. The question becomes, can a person maintain this lifestyle long-term? Because, unlike calorie counting, you can't necessarily take a vacation from it on the weekends and keep getting results. Low-carb dieting is dependent on putting your body into ketosis, and that doesn't usually happen overnight. When a low-carb dieter has a bad weekend and eats too many carbs, it may take a few days of being strict again before they get their body back into that ideal fat-burning mode known as ketosis. But, as with most things, people vary. Some people may be able to eat carbs on the weekends and have no problem continuing to lose weight. Some people may just not get the same weight loss benefits from a low-carb diet as others do. And some people, like me, just won't or can't eliminate something completely from their life. Or it may give them such an upset stomach that they can't leave the house (remember the chronic diarrhea?). Also, I found that at some point I just plateaued and couldn't continue to lose weight. Works great for some people! Don't know until you try, right?

How many carbs is right for me? Again, good question. And just like with calorie restriction, it is going to vary, not only from person to person but from plan to plan. Atkins, keto, paleo—all vary on how many carbs are allowed and will vary even more depending on how fast you want to lose or if you're strictly maintaining. If I have to hear about keto any more, I might scream, but without a doubt, people are finding success with it, and I say if it works, do it!

Where to Start. Atkins, keto, Dukan, low-carb paleo, low-carb Mediterranean, low-carb Whole 30, South Beach Diet, zero-carb diet ... just do a little research and determine which one works for you. Atkins has products in the store to help, as do some others.

Pros:

• Little to no calorie counting or food tracking necessary; just follow the rules and eat.

• It is VERY popular right now, so you can find tons of recipes and help online.

• Sit-down restaurants will make this easy ... steak, chicken, veggies, easy. You can eat a ribeye ... yummy fat.

• Ranch. Dressing.

Cons:

- You have to eliminate some things from your diet—white flour, white sugar, etc.

- Fast-food eating can get hard. Things get very limited and you have to get creative.

- Doesn't allow for mistakes; it's kind of an all-or-nothing situation.

CALORIE COUNTING

Why this works for us. This is as basic as it gets and really is at the heart of weight loss surgery. The point being that by eating less food, you lower your caloric intake and therefore lose pounds. This is an ideal place to start if you're trying to get back on track, because you're not having to completely eliminate anything from your diet. If you really want that Little Debbie Oatmeal Creme Pie, then you can have it; you just have to be smart about your other choices that day so you can fit it in. Not that a Little Debbie snack is a good food choice; I'm not advocating for it. I'm just saying that in the real world, we are often confronted with creamy delicious tempting snacks.

How many calories is right for me? Good question. According to my manual I got from my weight loss surgeon, I'm supposed to keep my calories under 1,000. Yeah, right. Here's the real numbers. I'm five three and 160 pounds. I have a good bit of muscle and I work out pretty hard four to six days a week. I have found that 1,200 to 1,500 calories is a good spot for me to maintain my weight. I have to keep it around 1,200 or under to lose any. According to standard mainstream medical advice, I need about 2,000 to maintain and 1,500 or under to lose. I can't say they're completely wrong, because here's the thing: the 1,200–1,500 limit is something I do on weekdays, but not on the weekends. No one is going to eat perfectly 100 percent of the time ... unless they're a robot. I am not a robot. I can eat fine during the week because I know that come Saturday, if I really want a little ice cream, I can have it. If I really want some ribeye on Sunday, it's fine. Saturday and Sunday, I do not track my food. I'm not a pig and I don't stuff myself, but I don't count all the calories. There are a ton of websites that will allow you to enter your height and weight and activity level and help you determine a good calorie goal for you. If you don't work out or work out very little, your number will need to be lower than someone who is very active. **My Fitness Pal** is an ideal solution because not only will it help you track your calories, it will help you figure out a calorie goal depending on how fast you want to lose, or if you only want to maintain your weight. It also allows you to put in your exercise for the day to allow for extra calories you burn.

Where to Start. My Fitness Pal, WW (Weight Watchers), Jenny Craig, Nutrisystem

Pros:

- Don't have to completely cut anything out of your diet.

- Pairs well with someone already limiting portions.

- Lots of programs to provide support.

- You can make it work when eating out if you plan ahead.

Cons:

- You really have to track your food and count those calories, which can get old.

- If you're used to ribeyes or ribs, things might get difficult ... sometimes.

- Low-fat dressing. Let's be honest ... it mostly sucks.

MACROS or FLEXIBLE DIETING

Why this works for us. We're getting a little off the beaten path, so I won't go deep into this, but this is something for people who really want to fine-tune their bodies or make sure their diet is balanced. Basically, it works like this: Food can be broken down into three categories—proteins, carbs, and fats. The percentage of each component varies depending on your goals at any given time. For instance, if you are wanting to gain some muscle, you will need more protein than someone who does not. More importantly in our cases, those who have had weight loss surgery want to make sure that their calorie intake isn't being overtaken by carbs and may want to set a particular protein goal to hit.

What should my macros percentages be? Like all things, it varies per individual and goal. The **My Fitness Pal** app allows you to track proteins, fats, and carbs along with calories. It lets you set percentages of how much of each you want. You would have to do some research as to how much protein is ideal for you but it should, at a minimum, make up at least 30 percent of your diet, and that is minimum. I shoot for 40 percent during the week and often fall closer to 30 percent, but I try, and trying is better than doing nothing for sure. Again, I try to hit this goal during the week, but on the weekends, I relax and enjoy life.

Where to start. The My Fitness Pal app, *Flexible Dieting Lifestyle* by Zach Rocheleau-(flexibledietinglifestyle.com), Lillie Loves Macros (lillieeatsandtells.com), Mason Woodruff (masonfit.com) ... Don't be scared off when you google this and see weightlifters or CrossFitters or other really muscled-up people. It is definitely favored by the very fittest people in the world, which means it can work for us too. These guys do this for a living and are what you'd call influencers, I guess. They are on Instagram and Facebook and they have websites and they come out with recipes constantly. They are also all very attractive and easy to look at, so there's that. I am sure there are tons more out there; these are just the ones I've come across who post consistently and offer really helpful advice, tips, and, of course, recipes.

Pros:

• It lets you take more control and really learn what your body needs.

• This eating plan truly promotes a fit lifestyle and helps tackle fitness goals.

• You can finally grow some abs, biceps, or the glute muscles that are so popular right now. (FYI, fat asses are in!)

Cons:

- More tracking required than even standard calorie counting.

- More of a learning curve.

- More planning may be required prepping food ahead of time.

- Less popular than other plans, so a little less info and pre-packaged food available.

INTERMITTENT FASTING

According to proponents of this diet, you're allowing your body to feed off fat stores during the times you don't eat. Again, this is a little off the mainstream, so I won't go deep into it, but if you like to skip breakfast, for example, or if you tend to only like a couple of meals a day, then maybe this is right for you. The general rule is you do not eat during a fourteen- to sixteen-hour span of time in a twenty-four-hour period (don't worry, this includes the eight-plus hours of sleep) and eat during the smaller eight- to ten-hour window. Whether it is because of my weight loss surgery or just my make up, I don't do well going that long without eating. I do get hungry, but more importantly, my blood sugar drops sometimes. I also don't enjoy skipping meals, so I never seriously considered this diet for myself, but it is an option to consider. This would limit your calorie intake if nothing else, and food tracking shouldn't be necessary.

Where to start. I honestly only have a little experience with this, and my research came primarily from Pinterest. Shocker. Have you figured out yet how much I love Pinterest? Seriously, though, I do suggest that you search Pinterest for tips and advice. The plan itself is pretty straightforward, so a few minutes of work should get you on your way.

Pros:

- Limited food tracking required.

- Limited food planning required.

- Easy to learn.

Cons:

- Probably will get hungry at first and will just have to suffer through it (LOL).

- May not work well for some people who have blood sugar drops when fasting.

- May not fit into your lifestyle.

PLANT-BASED DIET

I recently attempted this lifestyle primarily for health benefits. Meaning I didn't expect to lose weight, I just expected to feel better and try to avoid some health problems that come later in life (remember, I'm middle-aged at this point) like high blood pressure, cancer, etc. This is basically the fancy new version of being vegan, which means no meat, of course, but also no animal by-products such as butter, cheese, dairy ... It's not an easy lifestyle. I followed this plan for about four months, but only during the weekdays. I used a vegan meal delivery service because I don't live in an area with lots of shopping options for alternative diets and had very little experience with vegan recipes. Remember, I ate meat, butter, and cheese on the weekends. Here is what happened. I did actually feel better energy wise, which is great, but the gas that came from my body! I've already discussed my diarrhea, so why not farts? Again, I was told the gas would dissipate, but I'm here to tell you that it did not. It was terrible. I lost friendships over it. No amount of Gas-X or Beano touched it. Because of this, I felt bloated as well. Also, with my limited stomach size, I had trouble getting enough protein. It takes a lot more beans to deliver the protein of a few ounces of chicken. For that reason, my carbohydrate grams were way too high and I gained a few pounds in the process. Let's just say I went back to meat full time.

Where to start. The *Game Changers* documentary on Netflix and Purple Carrot (a meal kit delivery service). You can simply search "vegan" on Instagram, Facebook, or Pinterest and find tons of pages with recipes and advice. The *Game Changers* documentary got me really revved up about the benefits of eating plant-based because the film featured athletes versus hipsters (no offense, because I love a good hipster), and I figured if it worked for a professional weightlifter, it would be great for me. I loved the idea of feeling physically strong and full of energy. Included in the documentary was a visit to a firehouse where they convinced the guys there to follow the plan for a week, and a few had some DRASTIC drops in cholesterol and blood pressure during the experiment. I should say I researched and listened to the other side of the vegan argument, which is basically that (a) it's difficult to maintain, which is true, and (b) it's not going to give everyone the same results, which is also true. They also claim some of the research he presented could be misleading, but there were also many doctors on board backing him up. They claimed that if you want to be your healthiest and you want to have less disease, eat plant-based. It can actually ERASE some of the damage you may have inflicted on your body over the years. I do still love the idea of it, and I still try to work some of the healthy aspects into my diet by working hard to get more vegetables into my belly, because I find that they often get forgotten in my pursuit of that lofty protein goal.

Pros:

　　• May have great health benefits and help with disease prevention or reversal.

　　• May give you better performance when exercising or more energy overall.

　　• Animals don't have to suffer or die for you (just saying).

Cons:

　　• Difficult for those of us with tiny stomachs to reach a healthy protein goal.

　　• You may crop-dust unsuspecting people with your ever-present flatulence. You have to eliminate quite a few things from your diet.

　　• Eating out can be very challenging.

These are just the bare bones of diet plans. Within each category there are variations and subgroups. Not to mention there are diet plans out there that I may not even know about. I can't stress enough that there is no perfect answer here. The plan that is best for you is the one you are willing and/or able to do. Get excited about finding a plan. Do the research. Try something new. If it doesn't work, don't give up completely; just try another one. Try it a different way. Try planning better. If you can stick to something at least most of the time, it might be the plan for you. Everyone is going to have the occasional binge weekend. EVERYONE! You just get back on board and start plugging away. I don't care what anyone says, nobody sticks to anything 100 percent and nobody has the perfect answer. If they did, the world would be full of perfect people with perfect bodies, and the last time I checked, it isn't.

#

Tips and Tricks: Food

Protein Supplements

The best protein is from real food, but sometimes replacing a snack or meal with a protein bar or protein shake is great. Better that than a greasy burger or a bag of chips. There are a million and one protein options out there and I have tried them all. No, I really haven't. I've tried like eight, but when I find something good, I know it.

Protein Powder

This is the most affordable option. You need to look for one that works as a meal replacement for weight loss. It should be high in protein (twenty-ish grams per serving), lower in fat (under five-ish grams per serving), and lower in carbs. Nobody wants to use up their carbs for a protein shake. Also, I have yet to find a plant-based one that is as good as a non-plant-based one, so let me know if you find one. I prefer to use water instead of milk, and I like it chilled with a few cubes of ice. Buy a shaker bottle and go to town. You can even make fruit smoothies with added protein in the blender. You can also use the powders when baking for added protein. I have even used an unflavored protein powder that I added to savory dishes to boost the protein.

My recommendations:

- Quest
- ISO100 Hydrolyzed (the chocolate peanut butter one is the best)

Protein Drinks

Unlike powder, these are protein drinks that are ready to drink (no mixing required), so they cost a bit more, but they are convenient and probably the better-tasting option. Just like with other protein supplements, look for high protein with lower fat and carbs. These can be kept chilled in the fridge and are so convenient. If you like iced lattes, then these are a must-have. A large cup of ice, a couple of shots of expresso, then fill it the rest of the way with your protein drink of choice. Best three p.m. snack ever. Guilt free.

My recommendations:

- Premier Protein (caramel is the best!!)
- GNC Total Lean shake 25

Protein Bars or Snacks

These are great to carry in your purse or car in case you need a meal on the go. I don't eat them daily anymore because I've gotten burnt out, but after I take a break from them for a while, I eat one and find I like them for a snack and they help meet that ever-looming protein goal. There are also protein cookies out there. Be careful, because sometimes the calories on those can get higher than you would imagine and the carbs can get a little much, so read the labels and make sure they fit into whatever plan you are following. Also, there are protein chips. In my experience, many taste like crap. But I have found a few savory protein snacks that are edible and are definitely worth a try.

My recommendations:

- Quest Bars
- One Bars
- NutriWise Dill Pickle Krinkles
- Shrewd Food Protein Puffs (Brick Oven Pizza flavor rocks!)

Carbonation

Okay, I know your doctor said no more carbonation. But sometimes you just want a small soda and some bubbles. Like I said before, we live in the real world. First of all, never have it with a meal. You will be so uncomfortable because it just doesn't work. Maybe at your three p.m. break you opt for a small Coke Zero ... occasionally. Some things are more carbonated than others, and I find drinking carbonation straight from the container doesn't work. Once I pour it over ice, I can enjoy it a little, but it often leaves me feeling bloated, so it's a rare thing and shouldn't be a habit.

Vitamins

Even if you think you don't need it, keep taking your vitamins. My vitamin levels were being checked well after I stopped taking my multivitamin and they always came back normal, so I thought I didn't need them. I eventually started getting some mouth soreness, gum sensitivity, and general fatigue that we couldn't explain. Regardless of my levels looking fine on paper, they weren't. As soon as I went back to my multivitamin, B Complex, and vitamin C supplement, things went back to normal. Moral of the story; just take your damn multivitamin and avoid my mistake. If you start feeling tired, you're not going to have the energy to care about what you eat. If you feel good, you're more likely to eat right and get out there and exercise.

CHAPTER 5

MAKING A PLAN

Let's MAKE. A. PLAN.

So, we've talked about the mental aspect of weight loss, the importance of exercise, and the ever-crucial factor of food, including what we eat and how we eat it. Knowledge is great and valuable, but without a plan in place, it will only take us so far. So, let's make a plan.

First things first. We need to weigh and measure. It's not always fun, but it's important to keep track and write this stuff down. You need to see it. Without it, you can convince yourself you're doing great when you really aren't. Or you can convince yourself you're doing terrible when, in reality, you're actually making progress.

Weight

You really don't need a fancy scale that measures fat, body mass, and all that. They are nice, but fat percentages are a little hit and miss. Any old scale will work as long as you use the same one every time. My favorite time of day to weigh is first thing in the morning, before I eat, naked. Take EVERYTHING off. We all know that our weight fluctuates throughout the day, so choosing this time is ideal. It is the lowest your weight will be all day, so take advantage. You're usually getting dressed for work or for the day, so after you strip, step on and jot it down.

Measurements

We're going to focus on three basic measurements. Make sure that when you take these, you're wearing similar clothes each time. For example, if you're wearing a push-up bra on the first day you measure and then a sports bra on the second week, that's gonna be very confusing. If you're a guy, you still need to consider wearing clothes of similar thickness each time. My workout clothes tend to be snug and keep things in place, so I always measure myself in them. Tightness is important, because we all know that after significant weight loss things can sometimes ... sag a bit. LOL. It can make it hard to measure accurately, so the workout clothes help put everything back into place. The chest measurement is taken in the center of your breast. The waist is just above your belly button at the narrowest point. The hip is over your butt, preferably the largest part, if that makes sense. I tend to stand in front of the mirror while doing these so I can make sure I'm as accurate as possible. If you want to track other areas of your body, that's totally fine. Just jot your extra measurements in the margins. You could do your upper arm, upper thigh, or even neck. The three I suggest are the easiest to repeat without error and tend to be easy to measure accurately week after week. I have included a graphic to explain where to take each measurement.

On page 48, you will see a handy dandy sheet for tracking these measurements from week to week. If you would like to purchase the downloadable forms included in this book click on this link or go to etsy.com/baileybirdstories.com where you can find the worksheet packet that accompanies this book.

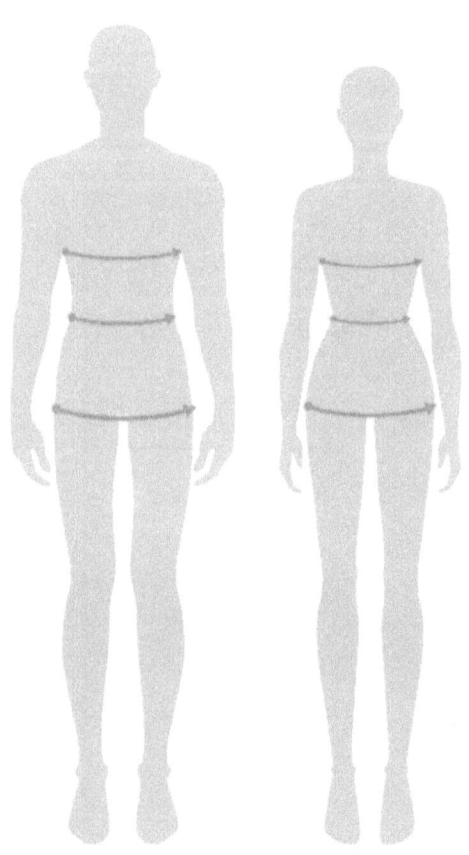

Illustration 175881381 ©ß Kateryna Golovchyn – Dreamstime.com

Weight and Measurement Tracker

Date: _____

Starting Weight: _____

Starting Measurements: Bust _____

Waist _____

Hip _____

Week 1 Results

Date: _____

Weight: _____

Measurements: Bust _____

Waist _____

Hip _____

Week 2 Results

Date: _____

Weight: _____

Measurements: Bust _____

Waist _____

Hip _____

Week 3 Results

Date: _____

Weight: _____

Measurements: Bust _____

Waist _____

Hip _____

Week 4 Results

Date: _____

Weight: _____

Measurements: Bust   _____

                          Waist _____

                          Hip   _____

Week 5 Results

Date: _____

Weight: _____

Measurements: Bust   _____

                          Waist _____

                          Hip   _____

Week 6 Results

Date: _____

Weight: _____

Measurements: Bust   _____

                          Waist _____

                          Hip   _____

The Six-Week Plan

So now we're educated on the basic pillars of weight management. You've been thinking about a food plan and planning an exercise routine in your head as you read along. I hope you're getting excited, at least a little. Now I'm going to ask you to do something that is going to shock you. I'm going to tell you pull back a little on the exciting plans you have in mind and take it slow. What?! The plan is broken down into weeks and this is an overview. Don't worry about memorizing or taking notes because there will be worksheets that outline and walk you through the next six weeks. I got you!

Mental Game

Weeks 1–3: Complete Nightly Planner

In the next section of the book, you will find all the forms necessary to keep you on track and prepared for the upcoming days, weeks, or months. The one you will use the most is labeled **Nightly Planner**. Get a stack of copies printed and put them on a clipboard by your bed. It is nice and short, so don't stress. You will just take a moment to note what went well that day and pause to consider what could make the next day better. You will also prepare for the next day by jotting down your plan for exercise and reminding yourself of your food goal for the next day. We're not attacking this thing all willy-nilly, so don't do it in the mornings, because they are just too hectic. Make these plans before putting head to pillow. You will go to bed all Zen and ready to kick ass the next day.

Exercise

Weeks 1–3: Twenty Minutes for Four Days a Week

I know it sounds crazy, but we're going to start small and build from there. You should be happy about that! For the first three weeks, we're going to establish a simple workout routine. Now, if you already have an exercise routine, then by all means, keep doing it. If it ain't broke, don't fix it. If you're already working out, then you're killing it and you're way ahead of the pack. If you've gotten out of a routine, no big deal. We're going to spend a few weeks developing a habit to build upon, so I've got you covered. If you pace yourself and follow this exercise plan, you will end the six weeks with a nice little habit. You can walk, ride a bike, do sit-ups, do kettle bell swings, play hopscotch ... it doesn't matter. As long as you spend twenty minutes devoted to any exercise of your choice, your task is done for the day. Just repeat it four more times before the week is done.

Eating

Weeks 1–3: Crucial Post-Surgery Habits Only

I know, this is crazy too. Not really, though. You have an amazing tool and you're going to use it to its fullest potential before you start eating boiled chicken and spinach for lunch. First, we're going to harness the power of the pouch.

Week 1: Eat slowly. Eat with purpose. Be thoughtful. Listen to your body. When you feel discomfort, even a little, stop eating. Get back in tune with your brain and your body. Quit allowing yourself to get too full. This is the beauty of a pouch. It is your new superpower, so use it. It also helps to use a small plate and only fix yourself appropriate portions. Your mother was wrong. You do not have to clean your plate! You can throw it away in your body or throw it away in the garbage. I would rather waste it in the garbage than waste it in my body.

Week 2: Along with eating slowly, you're going to add the habit of **no drinking five minutes before your meal, and no drinking until thirty minutes after**. Again, we're harnessing the power of the pouch. Don't flush that food out too quickly. We want it to stay and keep us full for as long as possible. It is not a difficult task if you decide to commit yourself. At the end of this week, you will have mastered two important habits already. Two!

51

Week 3: Along with continuing to eat slowly and no drinking during your meal, you're going to focus on **protein first** at each meal. This begins when you fix your plate. Remember to start with a small plate and only fix small portions. Focus on the chicken, the steak, and the meat, and have tinier portions of sides, especially if they are not vegetables. I'm still not asking you to drastically change your diet. Is the chicken fried? That's okay for now. Is the steak a nice fat marbled ribeye? I won't judge you. Also, I'm not saying you can't enjoy sides, but you should take two bites of protein for every one bite of a nonprotein. Focus on the protein! Three weeks out and you will have mastered the three crucial habits all post-weight loss surgery patients should have. Progress!

HALFWAY POINT … HOORAY!

At this point you are halfway to being back on track! The last three weeks should have been relatively easy, considering you didn't have to do a terrible amount of planning, you didn't have to change your food, and exercise didn't take away huge chunks of your time. And I can bet you lost a little bit of weight or a few inches. Even if it was only a small amount, how great to be able to have some success just by tweaking some small things in your life. Even if you didn't lose anything, it's truly not a big deal. If nothing else, surely you gained some confidence knowing you're back in control. If you completed your tasks even half the time you were supposed to, you do realize that you still improved from where you were. Better is better!

Now we're on to weeks three through six of the plan. It's time to take the training wheels off. I'm still going to be running behind you cheering you on, but you've got to take the wheel. You've got to start taking charge of your health. You're going to have to experiment, research, and try some new things. It is your journey, not mine. I gave you the tools and resources to get started, so let's get going.

Mental Game

Weeks 3–6: Complete Nightly Planner

Same sheet, same clipboard, same nightly routine for the next three weeks. Each night, pause before watching your recorded sitcom or passing out from exhaustion to fill in a few blanks of the **Nightly Planner**. Make note of what's working, what's not, where you can improve, and plan on that exercise. Plan your day, or your day will plan you.

Exercise

Weeks 3–6: 20___ minutes for 4 ___ days a week

Your initial goal of exercise was twenty minutes for four days out of the week. Notice that for the final three weeks, I've left some blanks. You need to decide if you want to stay the same or increase your exercise. You can't go backwards and do less, but you also don't have to make a drastic jump either. Take a serious look at your abilities and your time and determine what is possible. Also, beyond the amount you do, you also need to consider trying or adding some variety to your exercise. If walking does it for you, keep walking. Maybe try another path or trail. Do whatever works for you, but don't let it get boring. This is the time to focus on you, and with every session remind yourself that your body is important and should be taken care of.

Eating

Weeks 3–6: Crucial Post-Surgery Habits Plus a New Plan

For the second half of the program, you're going to continue those three crucial habits of slow eating, no drinking, and protein first. If you're progressing fine with those changes, you can continue with only those. Keep up the good work and use your pouch. If you need more to reach your goal, then it is time to determine which eating plan you want to adopt for a few weeks. If you have tried something before and found a good bit of success with it, try it again. If you want to try something new and start afresh, that's what you should do. Whatever you try, make sure to give it a fair shake before tossing it, but the fact is, the most successful diet plan is the one you are willing to follow. I encourage you to attempt the plan of your choice, the one you are willing to follow. I encourage you to attempt the plan of your choice seven days out of the week in order to get back on track. Nobody is perfect, so there will be some setbacks for sure, but trying and doing pretty well is way better than giving up. Once you reach the end of the six weeks, you can pull back to following a program five days a week and letting your hair down a little on the weekends. But for now, let's shoot for seven full days. That's why the program you choose shouldn't be so strict that you hate it. Choose wisely and don't be scared to try something new.

NIGHTLY PLANNER

"If you talk about it, it's a dream. If you envision it, it's possible. But if you schedule it, it's real." Tony

Robbins

What did I do well today?

1. _____

2. _____

3. _____

What would make
tomorrow better?

1. _____

2. _____

3. _____

Tomorrow is _____ **(Day of the Week)**

My Food Goal for tomorrow is _____

(food tracking, protein first, eating slowly, food prep, etc.)

My Fitness Goal for tomorrow is _____

(Wallking for 30 minutes, Pinterest workout, 100 squats, rest day, etc.)

What steps will I take to
achieve these goals?

1. _____

2. _____

3. _____

Weekly Goals at a Glance — Days Completed

			Days Completed
Week 1:	Mental Goal -	Complete nightly planner	O O O O O O O
	Exercise Goal -	20 minutes	O O O O
	Food Goal -	Eat Slowly! Stop at first sign of fullness!	O O O O O O O
Week 2:	Mental Goal -	Complete nightly planner	O O O O O O O
	Exercise Goal -	20 minutes	O O O O
	Food Goal -	Eat Slowly! Stop at first sign of fullness!	O O O O O O O
		AND No drinking 5 min before or 30 min after meal	O O O O O O O
Week 3:	Mental Goal -	Complete nightly planner	O O O O O O O
	Exercise Goal -	20 minutes	O O O O
	Food Goal -	Eat Slowly! Stop at first sign of fullness!	O O O O O O O
		AND No drinking 5 min before or 30 min after meal	O O O O O O O
		AND Protein First	O O O O O O O

Keep those **3 crucial goals** of EATING SLOWLY, NO DRINKING, and PROTEIN FIRST

Now its up to YOU to determine your EXERCISE GOALS and FOOD GOALS for the following weeks.

Week 4:   Mental Goal -   Complete nightly planner   O O O O O O O

             Exercise Goal - _____   O O O O O O O

             Food Goal -   3 Crucial Goals   O O O O O O O
                             AND
                             _____

                             _____
                             _____   O O O O O O O

Week 5:   Mental Goal -   Complete nightly planner   O O O O O O O

             Exercise Goal - _____   O O O O O O O

             Food Goal -   3 Crucial Goals   O O O O O O O
                             AND
                             _____

                             _____
                             _____   O O O O O O O

Week 6:   Mental Goal -   Complete nightly planner   O O O O O O O

             Exercise Goal - _____   O O O O O O O

             Food Goal -   3 Crucial Goals   O O O O O O O
                             AND
                             _____

                             _____
                             _____   O O O O O O O

CHAPTER 6

WRAP UP AND MAINTENANCE

You Kicked Ass!

Well, I'm impressed. By now, you should be well on your way to being a fit individual. You should now have the mental habit of planning ahead and tracking your progress. Very important. You should also have retaught yourself those three crucial habits that all weight loss surgery patients should have. You should also have discovered along the way a diet or eating plan that fits into your lifestyle and doesn't make you want to stab people.

This does not mean you are done. If only that were true. Before you get too carried away with yourself, take a moment to plan for the next week, or month, or year even. If you only had a bit to lose to get back to where you wanted to be, then perhaps you're ready for the Maintenance Plan, which we will be discussing in the next chapter.

If you have not reached your goal, no big deal. You've got all the tools necessary to keep on keeping on. You just have to keep planning and keep being accountable. Hopefully, you have a sidekick by now. Hopefully, you have an eating plan that works. Hopefully, you have a set of dumbbells or a gym membership to help you on the rest of your journey.

If you have more pounds to lose before you hit maintenance, the first thing I want to do is encourage you. Unlike so many people who want to turn things around or make positive changes, you did more than want it or complain about it or wish for it. You took action. You were not complacent. You know things don't just land in your lap. We have to go get them or make them happen. Congratulations!

How to Proceed Until You Hit Goal Weight

You need to keep your mental game high but pull back on the reins a bit with the strictness of your diet plan.

Mental

Keep doing the nightly planner form on weekdays only.

Exercise

Keep exercising just as you are now and try to shoot for the minimum of four days a week. That is what is going to be your reminder to take care of yourself, now and forever.

Eating

Stick to your eating plan as best you can Monday through Friday, but allow yourself some wiggle room on the weekends. On the weekends you can relax your food tracking and eat some yummy things that you don't allow yourself during the week (honeybun ... sigh), but the main habit you never, ever stop doing is the eating slowly rule. If you want to drink with your meals on the weekend at this point in your progress, go ahead. If you want to let that protein-first habit slip on the weekend at this point, go ahead. But I want to say again, no matter what day of the week it is—ALWAYS EAT SLOWLY! Use the power of the pouch every day of the week.

#

Maintenance Plan

Look at you! You're back at your goal weight! You kicked ass!

Now what?

Maintenance Plan

Now that you've hit your goal weight, you can relax a bit. You cannot throw all the rules out the window, though. You still have to eat slowly and listen to your body. Here are the rules I use to stay at my goal weight.

Weighing Daily

You should weigh every morning, at least on weekdays. If your weight is up more than a pound, do something about it that day. It's as simple as that and as hard as that. What I mean is that it sounds easy in theory, but following through is tough. Our weight fluctuates for reasons other than fat. Menstruation, constipation, bloating—all will push the needle higher, so you have to know your body and how it reacts to different situations. If in doubt, do something about it that day. Eat the chicken, drink the protein shake, skip that snack, don't eat the chocolate, pass on the chips, etc. Make the right choices until the scale is back where you want it. Worst-case scenario, you didn't need to lose fat but the scale was only up because of constipation. You do the work AND go to the bathroom and the next day the scale says you're a pound under your goal weight. This is no tragedy, my friend. You're ahead of the game.

If things start to slip ... and oh, they will. Holidays will come. Depressions will hit. Testosterone will drop. Menopause will creep up. All these things can throw us out of whack and force us to work harder. Fight the battle. Tackle it before it drags you under. Go back to weekdays of work and weekends of relaxing. Get those worksheets back out and plan another six-week cycle. Read the book again. Hell, buy another book from someone else if it motivates you and gets you back on track. Always be proactive in your own life. Don't ever be the person who complains about what life has handed them. Be the person who does something about it.

CHAPTER 7

FINAL THOUGHTS

I truly hope that you end this book on a more positive note than when you started. To imagine that someone out there got even a little bit healthier because of this creation just blows my mind and makes me a little giddy. When I finally decided to commit to gastric sleeve surgery, I didn't imagine myself giving anyone healthy eating advice. I just pictured them looking at me, thinking, "You took the easy way out. What do you know?" It felt like giving up in a way. I soon learned that I wasn't giving up at all. I was just taking a different path—a path that would finally get me where I wanted to go.

Since finally reaching my goal, I found myself contemplating and thinking about what was working for me and what wasn't. I was looking around at others who were succeeding and failing and trying to determine why. I was talking to them and finding out what was going on in their day-to-day lives. One of those friends who had gained a bit actually began to cry. She felt like a failure and asked for advice. She's one of the reasons I decided to put it down in writing. Not only did I hope it would help someone, I hoped it would help me to stay strong and have a plan to keep me on track.

My final advice is not surprising. It's about continuing to take action. Complaining and complacency are useless, boring habits that need to be tossed. When confronted with a problem, any problem, you should always do some thinking, do some research, and most importantly ... Make. A. Plan.

Link to Printable Forms

If you would like to purchase the downloadable forms included in this book go to etsy.com/baileybirdstories.com where you can find the worksheet packet that accompanies this book.

Make. A. Plan. /Bailey 84

www.ingramcontent.com/pod-product-compliance
Lightning Source LLC
Chambersburg PA
CBHW020617220526
45463CB00006B/2606